GREYED

GREYED

April Brewer

GREYED

© 2021 April Brewer

ISBN: 978-1-7350965-3-7

All rights reserved

For permission requests, email the publisher, addressed: "Attention Permission Coordinator," at the following address:

Samone Publishing

Drsamone2016@gmail.com

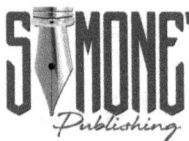

samonepublishing.com

ACKNOWLEDGEMENTS

I want to say thank you to all those who have supported me throughout my journey of life in helping me become the phenomenal lady I am today, whether you have been in my life the entire time or only for a season. I am forever grateful. The proceeds from this book will benefit in making a better life for myself and others.

I would like to give my deepest gratitude and say a very special thank you to my biggest supporter, my dad, William. Dad, you are the person who always knew I could do anything, even when I didn't think so. Without you I don't know where I would be today. Thank you for being the first to love me, being there for me and for believing in me through all my endeavors and failed attempts, even when I didn't believe in myself. Thank you for being my rock and teaching me strength because I am the strongest I have ever been to this day.

Also, to my friends, the ones who brought me groceries, supported my successes, took me to doctors' appointments and other places, paid my bills ,and pushed me to strive beyond my expectations to be the best person I can be. Just know I am forever indebted to you and forever grateful to have you in my life.

I am also thankful to all my friends who have supported me through other aspects in my life because I don't know where I would be without the love and kindness from you, I am forever grateful.

Love you all,

April

TABLE OF CONTENTS

PREFACE

WHAT DOES GREYED MEAN?

A very important person in my life told me that I see the world only in black and white. She told me I had no grey area in my life when it came to myself or receiving it from others in my life. She fussed and made sure I knew that everything was not always black or white, and instead of answers of yes or no, I should accept a maybe or a I don't know or something from people.

The reason is because things don't always go according to the way I want it to, and everyone doesn't always have an answer when I need it from them.

Also, when it comes to having grey areas in your life, it can be miles long, instead of a small area. So, this got my mind running and wondering, "How many things have I accepted or not accepted by not being grey."

I thought maybe this is how we should view race—everyone's nationality is Grey—we all bleed red blood and in viewing it this way maybe racism would be over. My mind wondered so much; therefore, how I introduce you to not only my black mind and not even my white mind, but to the new addition of my grey mind for my new grey life is the purpose of this book.

Also, I could have spelled it as Gray, but I like Grey better.

To anyone who has ever had a dream

that was hard to obtain,

never give up …

some dreams do come true.

To anyone who has had hard times,

please know things do get better.

Chapter One

RELIEF

The winds blow the trees as they bend further and further than their normal curvature.

The rain comes, the sky darkens, the mixture of them together makes it to where I can no longer see out the window.

The sirens go off like crazy, one after another, until they start to echo one another in the neighborhoods nearby.

I notice that the storm is close to me now, as my house starts to sway. I know a tornado is near. As I see swirls from my window, I head for the bathroom to emerge myself in the bathtub for cover.

The weatherman on the TV says the storm is in my area around my house. At this point, I turned the TV off because I didn't want to be afraid. I decided to stay calm and not panic. I was so calm until I fell asleep in the bathtub without knowing I did.

When I awoke, I expected to find a catastrophe and disaster everywhere. But to my relief, when the storm with the tornado passed my house, there was very little damage done to my house, and no damage to my car, which was outside. Thank you, Lord, for your protection. But, I did notice this wasn't the story for everyone around me. So, my volunteer nature kicked in, and I went to work helping others, letting them know that everything would be alright.

I knew that I was the joy from the storm, and I wanted to share it with others for encouragement.

There was cleaning, moving, packing, and restoring so that we may all start a new Chapter in life. Just to know that it was over now gave everyone the opportunity to take a deep breath. It was such an amazing feeling. A new start for all of us after the storm. What a relief!

And it was a relief to know that even in the midst of the storm, God was watching over us. In Psalm 121:5-8 we read, "The Lord watches over you—the Lord is your shade at your right hand; the sun will not harm you by day, nor the moon by night. The Lord will keep you from all harm—he will watch over your life; the Lord will watch over your coming and going both now and forevermore." (NIV).

Chapter Two

OBESITY

I eat to make myself feel better. I even eat when I'm not hungry. I sit and eat as I watch TV, not knowing that I am continuing to stuff my face without any hunger intention or even realizing that I have eaten a whole, big bag of potato chips, a sandwich, and a box of candy.

I've eaten and eaten until my body starts to ache and my bones can't handle my own body weight or the mass that I have now created.

I look in the mirror every day, and instead of seeing someone beautiful, I only see my fat. A big ole fat person looking back at me.

I tell myself that I will start the process of being healthy tomorrow—BUT tomorrow never comes. Instead, I'm back in front of the TV, watching my favorite shows and stuffing my face once again. The couch is my best friend. I go to stores and see millions of models on the magazine covers and make myself believe that I can be like that if I just work out, but I want to take the easy way out because I don't want to work out and sweat like crazy, why would I?

Really ... Why? Why would I do that when I can go and have surgery or some new technology procedure? I don't do it because I'm afraid that I might not make it out alive or look the way I imagine myself—all model like—whenever I go out in public. I get so anxious knowing that everyone around me is talking about me and my body and staring at me telling fat jokes.

I want to stop, but the food is just too good and the next thing I know is I am back on the couch. Even though I'm fat, I have feelings too. My clothes no longer fit, so I buy new ones, bigger ones. My doctor says my health is in danger, and I need to change my lifestyle habits, but why would I when I like my life? Why can't skin be skin, and we show how we are all shaped differently without being criticized. I mean you only get one life so why not enjoy it the way you want to—so I surrender to myself.

However, I also want to be good to me, and I know that includes watching what I eat. The Bible says, "No discipline seems pleasant at the time, but painful. Later on, however, it produces a harvest of righteousness and peace for those who have been trained by it" (Hebrews 12:11, NIV).

So, I will surrender to the Greater One instead, and believe He will give me the strength to be healthy.

Chapter Three

ROAD RAGE

The open road, a place where you go when everyone leaves. The place they sleep on, which is their second home to get on the road early in the morning while it is still dark. You get in the car and your happy and eager to get to your destination, until you get halfway there and encounter traffic with impatient people. As you draw near to the car in front of you, another car decides to jump in front of you, cutting you off, making you have to jump on your brakes.

At this point, you become immediately frustrated with this person's stupidity. You start pointing fingers at them and cursing or you turn on your bright lights and start honking at them. Or you think about wanting to throw something out of your car at them.

But, as traffic breaks open for a split second, the car that cuts you off throws something at your car, which causes you to almost wreck into someone, due to you losing control and swerving. This makes you become even angrier. Now you feel like taking action. You roll down your window and pull directly up to the side of their car. They pull over and so do you.

Now Ya'll are both angry, cursing each other out, so you decide to get even by kicking their car and scratching it, and you tell them you will hurt them worse than they could even imagine. To prove your point, you pull a bat out of your trunk along with a taser. You both end it, deciding not to call the cops because you both would go to jail—you probably more than the other driver because they think you are the main crazy one, especially when you're black and she is white, and she has no weapons.

So instead, you get in your car and drive away, but you are still angry, and you didn't notice that you're speeding so the cops pull you over to give you a ticket. You try to get out of it, but he's not listening.

So now, because you have to pay a fine, you are even angrier and your adrenaline is pumping. So you go to the gym to work out the adrenaline, and you vent to your friends until you worked out so hard that you dislocated your wrist 20 minutes ago, and now it is swollen, so you pop it back in place feeling no pain and now decide that you are calm now since you have hurt yourself and not the other person like you wanted.

If you have driven on the highways very much, road rage is fairly common. But usually this only lasts a few seconds or maybe minutes. Anger on the other hand lasts much longer and can have a powerful, negative effect on our bodies. When these kinds of things happen to us, we have

6

a choice. Will we let the temporary cause a permanent health issue? Not only in our emotions, but in our physical bodies, as well?

This is when we seek the peace of God. The Bible says that His peace passes all understanding. Philippians 4:7 states, "And the peace of God, which transcends all understanding, will guard your hearts and your minds in Christ Jesus." (NIV). It is especially, at times like this, that we need help in managing our thoughts.

It's important that we keep these thoughts in mind and choose to "let go." In the long run, no one should be able to have that kind of power over us and our thoughts. We can choose! And when we make the right choices, we can keep both the power and our peace!

Chapter Four

TALKING PEOPLE—
CRAZY or NOT?

As I awake each morning and I arise, I see a picture in the mirror of my disguise.

I often ask myself, "What it is I forgot!" I'm talking to myself—am I crazy or not?

I wonder what's in the future for today. I give thanks to my Father God Almighty as I pray. The future is never promised to or for me or you.

I follow the path that seems to lead me through and through trials and tribulations of what I seemed to have forgotten. Talking to myself, again—am I crazy or not?

The voices telling me to go left and right, my first reaction is to put up a fight, as I look at my torn clothes. I'm not ashamed. It's the crazy people in my life that I have to blame.

Every day as I walk down the street, I see people talking to themselves. So then, I often ask myself and wonder, "Why are we hearing voices in our heads? Is this a premonition of our past lives, trying to come back in the future from our endless cries, or am I insane?"

I'm also awakened at night with the terror of sweating and screaming. Is this a reality or am I dreaming? But, here I go again—the voices I have seemed to forget.
Am I talking to myself, am I crazy or not?

Is this a reality hidden so deeply within that the voices keep telling me we are only just friends, but maybe I'm not crazy, and it's just my intuition being jumbled together that is confusing me.

So, I ask this question to everyone: "What do you think, am I insane, crazy, or what?"

Maybe you have heard these same voices talking to you. Confusion is from the enemy. This is why it's important to know who you are and whose you are. The Bible tells us as children of God we have the mind of Christ. (1 Corinthians 2:16). This means we have the ability to stop the negative, unproductive talk with the Word of God, which changes everything. When we use the Word, peace flows, confusion leaves, and we can hear clearly now.

Chapter Five

MY UNSAID FEELINGS

We hang in a group, but never one on one, so instead, you embarrass me all the time because you are the one who is insecure. It's okay. I understand our situation, but sometimes you do not want to talk about it and that's okay, too.

You should have talked to me before you passed me in the group, so don't try to talk to me now. Think before you speak. If you were upset and you said you didn't want to talk about it as a friend, I would respect that and leave you alone and not talk about you behind your back. The most I would say is, "I hope she's okay." Why? Because I felt you went a little crazy, going on and on about all my faults because that's not what a true friend does. If you had a problem with me, you could've tried to talk to me on the side when the time was right and you could actually tell me what's up and give me whatever advice you felt I needed.

Even when I made multiple comments that what you were doing wasn't ok. Throughout this year alone, you said MANY insults: like I'm fat, I'll never get married, I won't find a prom dress in Ms. B's room, I won't make it in college, and other things, but guess what, I let them go, and those times I didn't cry about it. But, I never forgot. You don't know anything about me. You don't know my family, besides what you see. You don't know my extended family at all. You don't know where I live, what I've been through, what I'm going through, or who my friends are outside of school, you don't know ANYTHING besides what I told you, and that's just like 5 percent of my life.

Don't you DARE judge me or say anything about me when you don't know ANY of my testimony. Just leave me alone for that matter. You were never a friend, and not once have I heard you say one nice thing to me without following it with negative comments. You get one chance and one chance only because I don't have time for the foolishness.

It's so easy to smile when you're hurting. It's easy to fake it in public and sob once you close the doors and are all alone. But I refuse to let people who never rooted for me, never supported me, never loved me, never cared for me be able to take my happiness, my joy, my love for life, or my confidence. I am strong enough to handle what comes my way, but I'm also smart enough to let stupid stay with stupid. I know I'm a great person and an even better friend. Before judging a cover, read the book.

And the best book to read and the most sold book in the world is the Bible. The instructions to walking out a loving, forgiving life are made very clear by our Savior and Lord, Jesus Christ. When we follow Him, we can live a fruitful and productive life, regardless of who or what happens to us.

Trusting in Him is the best way to take your life off of the victim path and on to the victorious one He created for you. Proverbs 3:5-6 says, "Trust in the Lord with all your heart and lean not on your own understanding; in all your ways submit to him, and he will make your paths straight."

Chapter Six

LIFE

It starts the moment you are born into this world. Life. It is like an obstacle course. You can either be dealt a good life or a bad life. There are ups and downs that will make you feel like you're on an emotional rollercoaster. There are things that will throw you curveballs to try and hurt you, and there are things that will just try to distract you from your goal. There are huge ladders to climb and ropes to pull. The major key in conquering the beast named "life" is to be open-minded and keep your priorities in order. Because no matter what curve ball is coming your direction or how many people try to bury you alive, you will be able to use the strength that is in you to overcome any and everything.

Sometimes there are even more instances where you feel like there is no way out, and it feels like you have run into a brick wall. You then get knocked down over and over again, and you feel like there is no way you can win or make it through. However, if you put your mind to it and find a new strategy, there is nothing that can knock you down permanently. If you believe you can do it, you can. The key is to not let life control you, but you control life.

15

You will mess up a lot, but you will get the opportunity to start over again and again over time. Just know don't take life for granted and enjoy each moment because you never know if they will come again or to an end.

The lesson to life is to live, love and give because these are the ultimate secrets to being successful in this life. Live for what life is right now and the beautiful things it will give you in the future. Love everyone whether you are close to them or not or whether they treated you right or not because only you are in charge of how you treat people, and last, give.

Give to others not expecting anything back, but with the heart and the mindset to help those who have less than you. Because there will be times when people will need your help and give you nothing in return. It will be okay because someone else will look out for you later. These were the keys our Lord taught us.

The Father loved us so much that He gave His Son, and Jesus loved us so much that He gave His life to restore us back to the Father. When we love one another, we are obeying the plan of God—Nothing is more rewarding or fulfilling than that. John 13:34 states, "A new command I give you: Love one another. As I have loved you, so you must love one another."

Chapter Seven

THIS WORLD NOW

Fury just burns inside of me like an open flame. Why are people so arrogant? Why are people so ignorant? Why are people so angry? Why do we take issues and matters into our own hands? I don't know why. People just love to try to tear you down, I guess. You ask yourself, "What's wrong with me? What did I do to deserve this world? Do I deserve this?" It astonishes me how often I see this.

I ask, "Why do I keep seeing the same type of situations on the news? Why can't we learn from our mistakes? Why does race matter in this world today?" We have come so far, but we have fallen so far backwards. "What makes me, a little black girl, a human being, different than anyone else? Skin color?" Well that's weird.

Crayons come in all varieties. "But, what makes one crayon greater or less than the other? Its color?" As far as I am aware, they both can be used to create beautiful artwork. And, unless I'm mistaken, you cannot create art with only one shade of one color. Am I wrong? For the most famous artists, Van Gogh, Monet, and Da Vinci, all integrated colors of all shades to create their now world-famous artwork. "Why can't we do the same? Why can't we realize that every race plays a crucial part in what makes the world successful." Each culture is one crucial piece of the puzzle. Not all the pieces will match, but when we work together, we create a beautiful picture. A picture that will last forever and that will tell many stories forever.

The Bible has literally hundreds of verses that deal with love, happiness, unity and peace. We read in 1 Peter 3:8, "Finally, all of you, be like-minded, be sympathetic, love one another, be compassionate and humble." To be like-minded means to be unified.

Philippians 2:2 says, "… then make my joy complete by being like-minded, having the same love, being one in spirit and of one mind."

But one of the clearest verses is found in Colossians 3:14, which states, "And over all these virtues put on love, which binds them all together in perfect unity."

So, the question is, "How long will it take for everyone in the world to learn that together we are greater? Or how important it is that we walk in love toward one another?"

Our world can't heal without a little peace and love. Let's all try to do our part.

Chapter Eight

CONFIDENCE

You know what's funny? I felt like I was getting stuck in the same situation, kind of like Deja Vu. For instance, if I felt like I was doing something in the right way for once, someone or something always discouraged me, and I made a complete circle back to how I felt before—as a failure.

But something in me changed recently. It was a spark that made a fire burn within my soul and refocus my mind. I see a successful woman who is challenged everyday—not letting anything intimidate her, but letting the challenges motivate her instead.

I see men working in big businesses. They don't even break a sweat when something difficult comes out of the blue and they have to decide in seconds what to do about it.

I see teenagers of all shapes and sizes walk through hallways, not caring one bit about what others think about them. I so desperately wanted to be like them that I copied what they did and acted like others did not bother me. Sooner than later, I did not have to fake it anymore.

I woke up every day and looked at myself in the mirror and liked what I saw.

When I look in the mirror every morning and give myself a much-needed pep talk, I encourage myself to always do my very best. I walk with my head held high and stand tall as if no one else is taller than I am.

I walk into stores and smile at everyone, genuinely feeling good about myself. What people said or thought about me did not matter anymore, and honestly, it is the best feeling in the world. I finally can say I believe in myself, even when no one else does. I am bold and will not let anything or no one stand in my way. And I want to share my confidence with you.

One Bible verse that helped me with this kind of confidence was, "I can do all things through Christ Who strengthens me" (Philippians 4:13, NIV). Knowing you are a child of God, loved and accepted, regardless of how others treat you is a huge relief that will bring you comfort and restore confidence—even during a storm.

Chapter Nine

LOVE

Thank you for showing me what love is actually supposed to look like in real life, so that I don't compare myself to the things I see on TV and hope they happen for me, due to its fairy tale statue.

You said, "Love is: I feel like our heart beats are in sync; the one you can't stop thinking about day and night; because you wake up thinking about me and only me; you can't sleep without me when I'm not there with you; love takes care of me when I'm sick and vice versa. It compliments me, even when I look my worst. We complete each other sentences. When I'm falling, you run to catch me. When I'm in danger, you protect me. When I hurt, you hurt. When I cry, you cry, and we are bonded to one another forever. No one can ever take your place.

This love shown comes from your friends, your family, and those who come close to you. Even though we are all opposites in every way, shape or form, we still love each other, even through the different things and ways of life we experience. You push me to do the best for myself, even when I can't see it. You pray for me when I can't pray for myself. I can depend on you for any and everything I need.

It is an unconditional love. Just like the love the Father above has for us. It doesn't ask for paybacks, returns, or to do IOU'S. Love never keeps a count of wrongdoing. 1 Corinthians 13:5 states about love, "It does not dishonor others, it is not self-seeking, it is not easily angered, it keeps no record of wrongs."

Love is when we all grow old together being happy, even though we might get on each other's nerves every now and then.

It's hard work trying to work as a team, but we are a special team, and we compromise to solve the problems that life throws at us because we know that teamwork makes everything better. To each and every one of us that encounters love, just know being with you is like having a sugar rush. It's just so sweet!

Chapter Ten

ANGER

So, picture this: Yelling at the top of your lungs, eyes bloodshot red, screaming, crying uncontrollably, pain eating you up inside so much that it feels like someone is stabbing you to death. The raft burns inside of me, I see fire burning red.

Revenge is what I seek, and I'm so mad I'm already contemplating my revenge. I want to burn your things, I want to break your things, I want to punch you in the face, my eye twitches, and I want to make you just as upset as I am because you made me upset on purpose.

I didn't call me, you did. Because before I was even upset, I warned you to stop. You continued to say stupid things to make me even madder. The enemy, Satan, was in me at this point. Negative thoughts ran throughout my mind in order to find one to choose from. I am now destroying things by breaking and smashing them and throwing them at the wall.

I hear ringing in my head, my head pains and spins. I want to hurt you as badly as you hurt me, so you know what it feels like. I am ashamed to say I know you. I'm ashamed to even come see you alone, and you want me to bring people with me—no way! Why, so you can claim a witness? You brought this on yourself. You beat me with your words and objects I thought that was enough, but no, you use me as a setup that didn't stop you.

Listen, I don't tolerate`bad behavior because of my attitude. My eye twitches even more and more as you truly upset me. You've lied, slandered my name, tried to defame my character. If you are going to claim I said or did things, then let me actually give you what you are asking for because I'm not going out without a fight and I'm not going peacefully.

I don't like attending things that are in my neighborhood, let alone your neighborhood. I ask you one question, then you attack me, why? Because of power struggles? Is my anger worth it? So, don't cross this fire pit unless you want to be burned and don't light the fire, if you know you can't handle the heat.

When this happens, I have to ask myself, "Why? Why do I allow you to irritate me. Why?" Then I snap at others when they haven't done anything to me. I'm so mad I'm contemplating my revenge on you ...

Why must you always attack the people who love you the most. I know Jesus, and I go to church, but the worst thing you can do is make me mad. Jesus may be my brother, but Satan is right there to stir up the heat—stir up my temper.

Having an attitude isn't the answer, I know, but when we are hurting so badly, sometimes we try and tell ourselves, "I don't care. I'm hurting, so I want to hurt others." Truly, who knows how either one of us will react in situations?

Sometimes it only takes saying, "Sorry," for a person to let it go. Can we be the bigger person and be the first to apologize? Restoring peace in the long run is the best answer. James 1:19 states, "My dear brothers and sisters, take note of this: 'Everyone should be quick to listen, slow to speak and slow to become angry,...'"

For the sake of our own health, let anger go and allow peace to move in.

Chapter Eleven

DREAMS

Walk with me into a night of dreams. Where everything is not what it seems.

Like lollipops hanging from trees and candies floating downstream.

Like dancing and singing objects flying in the night. They're a figure of your imagination, but you see them in site, and everything is just carpe diem.

Walk into the light they say, but you decide to stay. I work toward endless dreams that can't be obtained in the ending.

I fail over and over again to try to reach the end. Like falling in love with a faceless man or falling off a building with no bottom, like a glimpse into your future and forgetting what you saw when you arise.

Or getting scratched up by cats, but to awake with no cuts, even reliving the past in order to correct the mistakes you once made, but to realize it's only a dream.

You see something bright, you walk into the light and boom, you will soon come back to reality.

I am the only one who can believe in me—myself—because I know God believes in me as His child. I know that I can do anything I set my mind to, because His Word says, "I can do all things through Christ Who strengthens me" (Philippians 4:13).

So, staying focused and determined and relaxed will help conquer any and everything, including these things we call dreams.

Chapter Twelve

LONELY

Sitting quietly, thinking, crying, in a room filled with things; yet it feels so empty. Wondering why my life had to be this way. Trying to keep myself occupied.
Longing for company or a companion, but not just anyone.

Someone who compliments me, and I compliment them.
I just want someone to love unconditionally.
I just want someone to talk to.
I just want someone to care for; and for them to love me as much as I love them. I don't want to be with friends, but oh so much more. Am I asking for too much? So, I see you flirting with me, but I'm not that interested and confused. Because I'm lonely, should I accept him ... maybe as a friend?

Now, I secretly think of you all the time, but I am afraid to tell you. I secretly have feelings for you because I don't want to change the relationship we have as friends. It is something I value, and I don't want to lose it by making things complicated. My thoughts race because I don't know if you have the same feelings for me and are hiding them for the same reasons, so you choose to be lonely as well.

I try to fill the gaps with other friends to hang out with, but they always bring you up and ask me, "Why aren't you together, which makes my heart long for you more."

I'd rather be lonely forever than to mess up our friendship.

Have you ever felt this way? We all at different times have felt this way. The good news is that we are never alone. When we have a relationship with the Lord, we know that He is always with us. His Word promises that He will never leave us or forsake us. (Hebrews 13:5).

So, when anxious or lonely feelings try to come, remind yourself of His presence and relax. The truth is, He is much better company than any one we know on earth.

Chapter Thirteen

DEPRESSION

The walls are closing in on me as I sit here alone rocking in silence. I feel like life is not worth living. No one wants to help me, as I cry uncontrollably. They say things will be okay, but I don't believe them because I don't feel that way.

Maybe I should take my life from this earth. Some days I feel like jumping off a bridge, or slitting my wrists, wrecking my car, hanging myself, overdosing, poisoning myself, or fighting with someone I know I can't win with.

In my world there are mountains with no valleys and there is no escape. There are no pills, no therapy, no person who will truly understand how much pain, hurt, and sadness I am in every day. I am not looking for attention or sympathy. I am looking for a way out, but there's no way, no exit, no light. I only see brick walls, closing in on me.

I am looking for genuine happiness, but I don't know where to find it—I need to go get help. I am looking and I have been looking. But I feel like I am in a maze with no way out. I start to rock, and I can't find any comfort in food, loved ones, or entertainment.

When I originally asked for help, no one would help me ... so why now? They say I'm crazy in this room by myself. They say I look sad, and when people ask me are you okay, I want to say "no," but instead I say "yes" because I don't want sympathy. They say they don't believe me, and I'm sad all the time, and that I mope around everywhere I go. They say I'm not normal, my actions are not normal.

So, I tell them I'm working on me, and instead of answering them, I press on. Pressing on is the key. Believing in God's Word is what gives me the power to press on. The Word is truth ... and when I feel down, depressed, or like giving up, I can turn to the most powerful weapon on earth—God's Word.

When I read verses like Jeremiah 29:11, "For I know the plans I have for you," declares the Lord, "plans to prosper you and not to harm you, plans to give you hope and a future," how can I not have hope? If the God Who created me has these kinds of plans for me, then who can come against me?

This is when I renew my faith and press on toward the gifts and calling He has for my life. I can and I will move forward.

Chapter Fourteen

COLLEGE

The place where life as an adult begins. The place where freedom begins. The pressure to succeed in trying to figure out what to do with my life—trying to figure it all out. Having to pay for college when it used to be free. College loans, credit cards at every corner, signing up, putting myself in more debt, and not knowing about it until after you graduate, and the bills arrive. I want to not have any debt, whether it's school loans, medical expenses, life bills, etc.

Professors, who only see you as an ID# and not as a person, because they have so many students that they lose their tests. They lecture you and expect for you to understand what they're talking about and don't want to answer your questions and there's no personal teacher, no one on one tutoring, only peer tutoring.

Am I supposed to know what they know? They have experience and I don't. They leave you to be responsible and to figure school life out on your own. I pay them to teach me, but am I really being taught by them or teaching myself with books.

Meeting new people who some will become lifelong friends for an entire lifetime, and some will only be in your life for a moment or a season—the banging super hype parties until the morning hours, making you late for class, having a hangover, no parents to tell you what to do, babies being born, seeing life differently being on my own, doing what I want to do and the people taking advantage of you, no protection or guidance.

I wake up late because I wanted to sleep in, not worried about chores on a Saturday, college football games, tricks of getting free supplies to get a credit card, doing other peoples' homework for extra money, learning things the hard way, and having to do work study programs.

They asked me, "Why do I work like I'm the last person on earth who's trying to recreate life and living?"

DEBT!

And because college made me and didn't break me by the lessons I learned, well, I know what I've been through and I have struggled so much that I want a change, and I want to start over new, and I want to be able to be worry free after I graduate.

As many have experienced, debt is a huge weight. I battled with it for a while, but now I have come to understand that I can cast my cares on the Lord. (1 Peter 5:7). When I do this I have His peace, which also brings His joy. Now, all is well with my soul.

Chapter Fifteen

DESPERATION

She looks around for someone, anyone who would give her the time of day. She was empty inside and she needed someone to fill in the holes that had been created in her heart. No matter what kind of attention they brought her, gave her, just being noticed meant the world to her. She wanted someone to help her in life and the affairs of this world.

Little did she know how beautiful she truly was. Little did she know how many boys noticed her but were too shy to talk to her. Little did she know how many prayers were sent by her family for her to be born, and how many prayers were sent to thank the One Who made her.

She harassed guys to like her, but there was no emotion attached. She harassed girls to be her friend, but they didn't care. While at her first college party, she came across a boy who noticed how beautiful she was and how equally insecure she was and took her for granted. She really wanted to be noticed, but she knew she had real worries to deal with—like not enough money for bills, not being able to manage her living arrangements, or travel arrangements on a daily basis, showing up to unwanted, uninvited events, so he could see you and people would think she was cool.

She goes to social media for any and everything and to vent. I need you to notice me, my heart and life yearns for your attention.

If only she could see the beauty in herself like others could and how strong she was to conquer this world on her own.

The feeling of loss for something that's missing is why I'm desperate and just want to be noticed.

Peer pressure can make us feel insecure, even anxious in many ways. However, God already knew we would have those moments. This is why He sent His Word.

In Philippians 4:6-7 it says, "Do not be anxious about anything, but in every situation, by prayer and petition, with thanksgiving, present your requests to God. And the peace of God, which transcends all understanding, will guard your hearts and your minds in Christ Jesus."

We can have peace in every situation, if we will turn our thoughts over to God. Our emotions will be healed, and our health restored. What a great promise!

Chapter Sixteen

BETTER DAYS

The affirmation of the world needs to be at peace and to have hope it will come again. Hopefully, one day sooner, rather than later. I know it's easier said than done, but instead of people just saying it, it needs to actually be put to use.

If everyone just got along and were not so selfish, there would be no more wars, no more sickness, no more tears, no more fighting, killing, or shooting, or dying. But we continue to fight about any and every little thing—like about who is right and who is wrong, when it really doesn't matter.

But why do I have to think about this? Is it because I'm terrified I will not wake up the next day? But instead of being negative, I think about how I don't look like what I have been through. And how we should want to leave a legacy for our future. My Legacy, your legacy, our legacy, should be memorable and hopeful with a splash of grace and honor.

What do you hope to leave behind? Have you thought about family traditions or heirlooms? Just as the world revolves, this world will once go back to its original state, and we will once again have peace of mind, feeling safe, roaming free, without a care in the world. I just want a better life. Is that too much to ask for? We have to want to have more. Don't you want to have more? It starts with you and me.

Black people should be supporting black people, but we tear each other down. We lie on each other when we should be building each other up. Why not take a lesson from the white people and build up each other's bank accounts for starters? Why not take a page from the Hispanics and support each other like a tightly knit family should be? More Sunday dinners, more movie night dates, more family reunions, more bridging the gap in between the different cultures so that we are one. Be Grey.

Stay the course and keep the faith, for better days will come again. The Bible says, "Without faith, it's impossible to please God" (Hebrews 11:6, NIV). Pleasing Him should always be a priority. Is it hard to use faith when you see the wickedness and evil that happens on a daily basis? Of course it is, but this is why it's so important that we each do our part to walk in love and support one another, regardless of color or creed. When we let the love of God shine through us, we will not only be changed, but so will those around us.

Chapter Seventeen

LIES

Why lie when the truth will set you free? Just so you can make yourself look good, just so you won't get into trouble. Instead, you blame others because you don't want anyone to know the real you. Is it because you know you did something bad, or is it because you just don't care? Maybe it's because you think your life is better than everyone else's.

Or is it because you really want to take that one secret with you and keep it to yourself? Or is it because you have done it so much it is now second nature to you to lie? Or is it because you think you're better than others? Or is it because you can get away with any and everything you want … maybe even murder?

I just want to know the answer to this question. Why lie when the truth will set you free? Why lie in order to try to hurt someone else? Did you even think about what that other person is going through and how your lies might affect them?

It's like when you are talking about someone behind their back, and they hear you. Once they ask you about it you say, "Oh, I didn't say nothing." Why lie when you got busted?

I'm shocked that you still chose to lie as if you weren't heard. Please know you will be the one paying for it in the end while you are trying to cover up what you did. Lies always come back to haunt you. Why? Because you tell one lie after the next, and after a while, you don't even remember the lie you told before. There is no need to lie.

The Bible has over 100 verses that deal with lying. Here are just a few. After reading these, I'll let you decide whether or not telling the truth matters.

"Truthful lips endure forever, but a lying tongue lasts only a moment" (Proverbs 12:19).

"The Lord detests lying lips, but he delights in people who are trustworthy" (Psalm 12:22).

"No one who practices deceit will dwell in my house; no one who speaks falsely will stand in my presence" (Psalm 101:7).

"For, Whoever would love life and see good days must keep their tongue from evil and their lips from deceitful speech" (1 Peter 3:10).

"Save me, Lord, from lying lips and from deceitful tongues" (Psalm 120:2).

Chapter Eighteen

MONEY—GREED

That green piece of paper that makes the world revolve. Or so they say. It's the root of all evil.

It's the reason why friendships and relationships end or get worse.

It causes trouble as soon as it comes into your hands or the other person's hand.

It's something people expect you to pay back, and when you don't, all hell can break loose, especially when you say you're going to "borrow it" because that insinuates payback.

It buys things that are not good for your health or that can put you in jail, like starting businesses with people you think you can trust, and they steal from you.

It wrecks us emotionally because we work hard for it just to end up giving it away to someone else.

For what?

We kill for it. We fight for it and over it.

Yes, money makes the world survive, but honestly how much of it do you really need? Be satisfied with what you have. How do you know how much is enough when you need to pay for things? Being money hungry will wear you out and make you so tired and exhausted you won't remember what you did yesterday.

You lose friends, you're lonely, your world is only about you, and being greedy gets you killed, especially when you flaunt your wealth.

So, I say, let the greed go, and use only what you need!

The Bible says in Mark 8:36-37, "What good is it for someone to gain the whole world, yet forfeit their soul? Or what can anyone give in exchange for their soul?" The soul is our mind, will, and emotions. If we lose our mind, will we go very far? ... Probably only to the hospital.

Greed can be a driving force, and it's not a positive one. So, rest in the Lord. His Word promises us blessings— health and provision. Maybe it's time to chase after Him, instead of money?

Chapter Nineteen

SCARED

I'm in a big house all alone. There are huge windows with no curtains and small windows with blinds. Just too many windows in this house, and I feel like someone is watching me with every step I take.

I hear noises, howling, bushes rustling, cars passing, knocking coming from somewhere, but in the place, I cannot find, I can see lights flashing in different areas.

Trying to stay calm. I try to fall asleep, and it is hard because I feel like someone is going to come out to come and get me.

Once I doze off, I keep jumping out of my sleep because things are distracting me.
I dream a cat is scratching me up.
I dream the alarm system is broken and someone is
      breaking in.
I feel a tightening in my chest and a tickle in my throat.
I feel like my body just split in two.
I feel bugs crawling on me everywhere.
I'm sweating profusely—it's so hot.
I'm falling off a building.
Getting beat up by a stranger.

I just found out my friends died.
I am terrified.
Will this nightmare be over?
I lift the covers higher.
There is no one to help me.
I just want to be set free from this scary nightmare.

I awake to realize I was never alone and had no reason to be scared.

This is the comfort that a relationship with the Lord brings … we are never alone. The Word states, " Be strong and courageous. Do not be afraid or terrified because of them, for the Lord your God goes with you; he will never leave you nor forsake you" (Deuteronomy 31:6).

Fear is of your enemy—the devil. Faith is of God. Faith comes by hearing and hearing His Word. Faith allows us to trust God and be at peace when we are going through difficult or trying times. And His Word is the source that brings us His peace.

Chapter Twenty

PANIC

You see a truck on the wrong side of the road heading your direction. You only have about two seconds to make a decision before you both crash into each other.
This is a one-way street, and you only have woods on one side and a wall on the other. All your senses and major decision thinking are all jumbled up into one.

You know you can't think, but you need to take some action. You try to hit the brakes, but the car doesn't stop. Your brakes have now gone out, which is now another problem.

You try flashing your lights, but he doesn't stop.

You really need to think, but you can't, and you start to cry because you see your life ending.

There is no time now to put the car in reverse.

What would you do?

My body hurts. I can't think or remember anything. I only see black.

I hyperventilate. I turn the wheel to the left and hope for the best.

I faint.

I hear people talking, but I don't see anyone.

I can't seem to pull myself together. I can't feel anything. Moments later I see lights flashing in my face, but it is still dark, and I feel as if I'm floating. When my eyes open, I see my car wrapped around a tree. I see the trunk on its side.

I panic—I scream. Loudly. What happened? How? Where is the other driver? I cry. I can't breathe. I can't think. I try to move … but can't. Wishing someone would please help me. Tell me.

There are people everywhere. I see them, but now I can't hear them.

I think how I want this nightmare to be over, but it is just beginning. I wish it had never really happened.

Many of us have found ourselves in accidents or other life-changing events and wonder, "Why? Why did this happen to me? What did I do to deserve this?"

It's during these times that we have to remind ourselves we have any enemy that came to steal, kill and destroy us. The fact that we are still alive is solely by the grace of God. He has a plan for us, not to harm us, but to give us hope and a good future. (Jeremiah 29:11).

When devastating things happen, we have to remember, even though it may appear in the natural that we are victims, the truth is we are and always will be victorious in Jesus Christ.

To God be the Glory!

Chapter Twenty-one

HARD WORKERS

Some of you wake up every day to go to a place of work in order to make ends meet when it comes to bills, kids, or even unexpected surprises. You work endlessly until you're so tired that you just pass out on the couch instead of going to bed like normal people.

Some of you work at a job that you should have teamwork on; yet they leave you to do everything yourself.

You leave work to go home and do more work because you have deadlines you need to meet and a family to take care of, so now not only are you still working for your job when you get home, but you need to do things for yourself and your personal life, as well. So, this makes you even more tired, and you feel like the work will never end.

You are so tired you don't even remember what you just said to me—let alone what was said to you. Even when the weekend comes, you have things that other people have signed you up for, making you still have the opportunity to not get any rest, along with adding that you still have things you didn't finish for yourself.

You try to make time for yourself and go to hang out with friends, but then they ask you for help with something, which makes more work for you.

The question is: When does it end for you? When is enough ... enough?

And this is what you constantly feel like. You feel like there are just not enough hours in a day for you to get things done, but only if there were 28 hours in a day, so that you could get just a little more accomplished or rest. You're running off of adrenaline every day, acting like a walking zombie.

To the hard worker's family and friends, just know it's not that we don't want to spend time with you or don't like you at the moment. It's just that we have goals that we want to achieve and obtain for ourselves, which has nothing to do with you. So, don't take it personally.

Some even work two and three jobs and/or go to school, living paycheck to paycheck, bill to bill, just to try and figure out how to get ahead and still manage to find time to be with friends, family, and have some alone rest time. But let's not forget about those sudden surprises that keep popping up in life.

Sometimes, you just honestly are so busy trying to meet the goal you are trying to obtain in your own life that you have no time for anything or anyone else, which is okay, because if they are patient enough, they will be able to be there during the payoff celebration of all your hard work.

So what do hard workers do when you have literally run your body down and you're so tired that your doctor says you have to quit doing something in order for your body to function for survival?

It's Wednesday, and I'm already tired, but my hustle will never stop. Why? Because "I can do all things through Christ Who strengthens me" (Philippians 4:13). And I have the Holy Spirit to lead me and guide me into all truth, which gives me the wisdom to know what to do and when to do it. This prevents me from overdoing it in areas and at times when I should be resting.

Jesus said to cast our worries on Him and to not worry because tomorrow would have enough worries of its own. (Matthew 6:34; Psalm 55:22).This means we take it one day at a time—letting Him lead us so our path will be easy and peaceful in every area.

Chapter Twenty-two

RELIGION

The space where you go to find peace from the physical world we live in.

This is a family, not a corporation space.

Where we all believe in the same God, and you should come to worship and praise Him for what He has done in this world, and yet, you think this is a place for you to put on a show and make yourself the center of attention.

This is not all about you because if it wasn't for Him there would be no you.

He died for our sins; and yet you sin in His house. You get upset, you curse and scream. At this point, you look to be on the devil's side by your actions.

You want Jesus as your Father, but you let satan be a close relative, too. This is not a Christianity versus Voodoo type of situation here. Are there consequences and struggles with your rituals between God and the devil? Sure there are. The curse is within yourself.

The church, the place we go to, is a hospital, a Godly hospital, but it starts within you. There's no judging, only a place to heal. Don't wound me in a place where I am supposed to come and be healed. In church you are supposed to be showing me love.

If you don't believe for you, no one else can. I feel bad when I am not able to worship, but I know the church is just the building, and I carry the church within me everywhere I go, because I am a God-fearing woman. A woman who is after God's own heart. A heart that I feel like is molded from gold, so I urge to have that heart of gold for my Lord and Savior.

I thank God daily. And you should too. Even though He is someone I haven't ever seen, I still believe. "In everything give thanks in all circumstances; for this is God's will for you in Christ Jesus" (1 Thessalonians 5:18, NIV).

How big is your faith?

If something major was to happen in your life today, how would that affect you? Could you still give thanks?

Start by learning how to change you, read your Bible, and then lead by example.

Chapter Twenty-three

ANXIETY

I don't know what happened to make me feel this way constantly. I used to not care what people thought, what people said, if they did not like me. Now, I cannot sleep at night knowing that the one girl does not like me.

I know she is a hater, but she continues to try to irritate me daily on purpose. My anxiety increases every time I see her come my way. Her personality comes in different forms, this I know. She says bad things about me that aren't true—behind my back and to my face. She now has a posse to talk about me to. "They tease me because I'm different, but I laugh because they are all the same."

On top of that stress, I have a major test coming up that I have studied my behind off for, staying up late hours tossing and turning some nights. And I can't focus because of her.

I feel uncomfortable the times I see her. I think the best way I heard it described was me feeling blind. I can't breathe. My thoughts get the best of me as my mind races. I do want to tell her off. But?

Sometimes, I think my own thoughts may have caused my anxiety to flare. I hallucinate because I feel like someone is following me or being watchful of things that are on me or being thrown my way, like a cat chasing balls. I feel there are plots being set up against me.

My heart races every time. I fear they will kill me by teasing me with things I'm allergic to like putting peanuts in my lunch. People talking to me, asking me questions, making me more anxious, nervous. I'm about to panic and cry.

I'm dealing with a lot that people have no clue about. I have to deal with high school antics from adults. I can't shake this feeling I have. Full-blown anxiety attack in full effect.

Regardless of the issues, at times, we all have to deal with feelings of anxiety. So how do we get things—the truth—back into alignment? Well, the first thing to do is just STOP! Stop and take a deep breath.

Then remind yourself about how much God loves you and the great plan He has for your life. The Word tells us that every good and perfect gift comes from the Father above. (James 1:17). You are His child. So, it doesn't matter who on this earth likes you and who doesn't.

He always works things out for our good. And if God is for you ... who then can be against you? (Romans 8:31).

Chapter Twenty-four

DENIAL

I sit and watch as things happen around me because I want to be aware of my surroundings. On one particular day, I sat in a friend's house. We watched as the activities took place with the neighbors, and we came and told others, but they refused to believe us.

People are not the same as you or me, and people are not all angels, as you might think. You refuse to believe the only person who would never lie to you. You say you know better, and that this can't be true.

You don't want to take responsibility for someone else's actions. But who said you did? People have helped you, and you say they didn't; you say you did it on your own. Lies. I know you don't really believe that.

Just like I know you stole from me because I set you up on purpose one day. I placed the money in the exact place I knew you would look—the exact spot from where you stole it before.

So, you just go ahead and act like nobody can tell you anything. That everything I say is wrong, and you say the exact opposite of what you think happened.

Your fan club, who you have wrapped around your finger, fed you the same lies you feed them.

Do you like it when they lie to you?

Stop denying the facts and the truth. For once, just listen and be honest with yourself.

Even the world has a saying … "Honesty is the best policy! If I lose mine honor, I lose myself." William Shakespeare.

Thomas Jefferson penned, "Honesty is the first Chapter in the book of wisdom."

God commanded us in the 9th commandment to not lie. Exodus 20:16, states, "You shall not bear false witness against your neighbor."

I admit, it takes courage to tell the truth at times, but in the end, it is so worth it!

Chapter Twenty-five

ANNOYING PARENT

All I want to do is enjoy myself, but my parents are always bothering me and getting on my nerves. They are always asking me to do things that I don't care to do.

As a child, my mom and dad had the freedom to do whatever they wanted, but they didn't always make the right decisions, and they feel like they missed out on some very good opportunities for themselves. Why do you speak negativity into my life?

Why do you get angry when I don't do what you want me to do? Why do you make it seem as if I have no life experience myself? Why is it that you feel like you have to tell me what to do about everything all the time, as if I can't learn on my own?

I hear you talking. I am listening, but what you need to know is that I have to figure things out for myself within my life. You have had your chance to live your life and you can't relive it through me.

Allow me to learn on my own and make my own mistakes. Why do you think that there is no one else in this world that I can trust but you?

How about the advice you give to me might be more appreciated if you said it in a different tone and matter of words you use?

You want to go where I go, know all my business, and want me to do the things you like when I want to do something different. I just want to know—can you just let me go? I want my own life to myself. Not your life through me.

Please let me go, because even though you annoy me, I do still love you. I'd just rather do it from afar.

At times, our parents can be one of our biggest hurdles, but I'm reminded that we are instructed in God's commandments to: "Honor your father and your mother … so it will go well with you" (Exodus 20:12, NIV).

Yes, they don't know everything, but there are still respectful ways we should deal with these situations. I want it to go well with me, so this is what motivates me to keep things honorable in my talk and actions toward them.

Chapter Twenty-six

SICKNESS / DISEASES

If I get bit by a bug there is a possibility I'm affected with a disease. At what point did bugs start being the source of infections and diseases?

We struggle and don't understand what's happening, not knowing what the outcome will be and having the "why me" syndrome. No one can help us.

Your body has taken over a new life of its own. The more you fight, the weaker you get, the tears, the pain, the negativity, the irritation, the memory loss, the traumatization.

Don't fight like you're sick; fight like you are a survivor; fight like you are already healed.

If you eat something wrong food wise, it's possible you may be infected with salmonella or listeria. Why?

If you go outside and the weather doesn't agree with you, you may get infected with the flu, cold or some virus, causing you to sometimes struggle to breathe.

Don't fight like you're sick; fight like you are a survivor; fight like you are already healed.

You didn't tell me you were dying or that you were even sick.

But you're here now ... claim it, you won.

We just want a better, easier life.
We are warriors, survivors. Take heed.
We want more freedom. We want more healing.
It may not come that easy, especially when people look at you in disgust, saying nothing is wrong with you.
Sometimes, I wish people would just mind their own business because we don't have to look like what we've been through.

Take me for instance.

Suddenly we become chronically ill, needing an emergency surgery and have no money to pay for it because we work at a job that paid below the poverty level. I had to be convinced to ask people for help or fight for my life—not knowing what tomorrow would hold.

What I would have liked to do is be able to say, "Okay, I'll pay for the surgery, and let's do it tomorrow!"

There were countless doctors' appointments, therapy, blood loss, swelling, and hair loss. I lost my home; my car had just broken-down months before, and I had a brand new car note.

I would like to say I'm going home to my own house and not to my parents' house with my bed on the floor. I won't be able to afford the medicine I need to control my many health disabilities. So, now I have to avoid certain things. I now have a new change of eating that I have to follow.

I want to be happy, and the only person who can see me get there is ME (and God) because I knew what I wanted. I didn't fight like I was sick. I fought like I was a survivor. I fought like I was already healed. Surgery did help me.

I come today saying I am in remission and free from all that has passed through my body in Jesus name.

I stand strong. I stayed in His Word. Why? Because the Words says, "He sent out His Word and healed them; he rescued them from the grave" (Psalm 107:20, NIV).

Please know that if you believe, your life can and will be changed forever.

Chapter Twenty-seven

FEAR

I'm a black sheep in a herd of white. I see the world differently. I'm different—I know—and I don't fit in one specific slot. I fit in several. Actually, I may fit in too many different slots. No one understands me. But I like it that way. My heart is racing, and it is about to jump out of my chest.

Because people are always attacking me.
I'm afraid of any and everything.

I sometimes fear my own dreams because the nightmares I have seem so real.

I also can be afraid and in fear of myself, because when I look in the mirror, I see my own worst enemy. Especially if I become angry and it gets stuck inside of me and I can't get it out, then I can't calm down.

I fear going to the country, because when I'm in the woods, it is not my friend at this moment. I mean it gets really dark.

I fear itching and scratching because I feel like something is crawling on me. Am I just hallucinating?

Even so, I think I'm going to scratch my skin off.
I fear things that move.

No courage doesn't live here, only fear! Or that is how it seems anyway, but then I am reminded of the Word of God which says, "For God did not give us a spirit of timidity or cowardice or fear, but [He has given us a spirit] of power and of love and of sound judgment and personal discipline [abilities that result in a calm, well-balanced mind and self-control]" (2 Timothy 1:7, AMP).

So, when fear tries to talk to me, I talk back with the Word and remind myself that God is always with me, leading me and guiding me, protecting me. After all, He did give His angels charge over me to protect me. (Psalm 91:11-12) Now, I manage my thoughts and peace comes over me.

Chapter Twenty-eight

EUPHORIA

I think I am smart ... and I know I am smart.
I am motivated to do so much.
I was told that I am perfect, that I can do anything.
I have been programmed this way.
I get $5 for ever 'A' I make, $3 for every 'B' I make,
and nothing for C's and D's.

As I increase in grades, the money amount increases as
well. You know extra credit. This is to help motivate me
to do even better.

I love my computer and books, and they love me back.
I love my computer so much that it interested me into
loving technology, period.

I take things apart and put them back together to challenge
my mind.

I apply myself to everything I do.
I am a part of multiple clubs and organizations.
I study a lot.
I think a lot.
I'm an overachiever.
I think outside the box.

I research a lot.
I can solve any puzzle you give me.
I get acknowledged for my accomplishments, and it makes me feel empowered. I have all these medals and cords, but what do they actually mean toward my smartness. A lot.

How have I made it this far? Hard work.

I see successful people doing well, and I transpire them to fit my way. I am different. When people talk, I understand them; but yet, they don't understand me.

Is it because my intelligence level is higher than theirs? I have people in my life who are way smarter than I am (mentors) and I have those who I wish were smarter (haters). But the question is: Am I as smart as I can be? No, I'm always willing to learn more.

When the Bible tells me in 1 Corinthians 2:16 that "I have the mind of Christ," I know I have the ability to learn and apply myself to an even greater sphere of knowledge. This also gives me the ability to do all things through Christ Who strengthens me. (Philippians 4:13).

How can we lose with Him on our side?

Chapter Twenty-nine

REMEMBER WHEN

Remember when men use to ask women out on a date?

Remember when guys use to open the door for us women?

Remember when they used to wine and dine you, pick you up for your date, and even ask your parents for permission first?

Remember when you first fell in love?

Remember when kids weren't disrespectful, and the only choice we had was to play outside, and when we came back in, we had to make sure not to let the flies in?

Remember when there were no diseases?

Remember when families stuck together?

Remember when you weren't scared of anything?

Remember when life was simple in certain times?

Remember when we all got along better than we do now?

Remember when it was against the law to break the law, and you paid for it?

Remember when there were others to help you through anything?

Remember when you wanted to grow up so fast as a child and be an adult?

Remember when you became an adult and you wanted to go back to childhood?

Remember when we laughed more than we cried?

Remember when there weren't so many rules to follow?

Remember when you could trust anyone to watch your children?

Remember when you thought your parents or grandparents were superheroes?

Remember when you thought you were grown and now you wish you weren't?

Remember when you thought you were rich and went on vacation and came back broke.

Don't forget the memories. They will last forever.

And don't forget to give God thanks in all things, for this is His will for your life. (1 Thessalonians 5:18). We know that not all our circumstances were His will because we have an enemy, but regardless, His will is for us to stay grateful and keep our heart and attitude right by giving thanks in all things—not "for" all things, but "in" all things. A grateful heart will keep us healthy and on the right path with the Lord.

Chapter Thirty

BROKEN FRIENDSHIPS

Your opinions are unwanted and sometimes should be kept to yourself. I keep my unsaid feelings balled up, which turns into more balled-up feelings than I originally had.

Why do you act bipolar all the time? Is there not any normal, full days with you? You are always late, and on your phone, and you take advantage of the niceness people are giving to you—you are actually being disrespectful.

So you forget my birthday, and instead of saying that, you lie to me, and over time, when I ask you, "Are we going to celebrate?" you feed me another lie on top of the lie, until I realize the game you are playing.

A lie you tell to me is the biggest mistake you ever made with me because I'm done with you after this point. I would never lie to you—let alone forget your birthday. And if I did, due to life being busy, I would do everything in my power to make up for it.

This world doesn't revolve around you, and it's not always about you. You can't continue to take and take from me and drain me of everything I have and not give something in return to make me feel that I'm valued by you, as you are supposed to be to me.

You say that I only do things that are important to me, or I only do the things I want to do, and not show up to all the things people invite me to. Well let me say this, if I feel like I'm unappreciated, why would I show up to something you invite me to when I know I'm going to be miserable and not enjoy myself? I have all of these negative things that float around in my head that I want to let you know and say to you, but I'm not that person, and I don't allow negative things to come out of my mouth.

I don't trust you anymore. You are supposed to be the one who knows me better than anyone else. So, I don't understand what made you think I wouldn't figure it out that you were lying to me. You should have known better because if I can catch a man cheating on me by seeing through his lies, what made you think I wouldn't see through yours? Is it because you thought since you weren't a man it would be different, or did you think I wouldn't care?

So, I'm just not that important to you, and I'm not going to continue to let you hurt my feelings. Yes, you hurt me. To be honest, this isn't the first time you have hurt me, or I have been upset with you and didn't tell you, but this will be the last time I feel mistreated by you. I no longer need a friend who is not a friend back to me. You are never there for me when I need you the most. When we spend time together it somehow always ends up being about you, and at times, you have left me there to go with some of your other friends or a guy, like we didn't come together, as if I didn't already drive far enough just to come and see you to watch you disappear.

I should have known better because I have seen you lie to your other friends before, but I thought it was different for you and me. Honestly, I thought to myself that we were more than friends, but that we were family, but I guess I was wrong.

But I love you enough to give you your space to live your life, and I love you enough to let you go so that you may grow. AND ... I love me enough to keep my mind in peace and for me to be happy. The Word says to forgive those who have offended you, and this is what I've done. Because I forgive you and love you, your offense won't steal my peace or joy. The joy of the Lord is my strength. (Nehemiah 8:10). And I want and need all the strength I can get.

Chapter Thirty-one

CLOWN

Do I amuse you with my silly antics, my off the wall craziness? Is it because I like to keep smiling? I sing and just keep smiling?

People say laughter is the best medicine. I bounce all around like I have ants in my pants and dance. I just can't keep still I have too much energy, like I ate a pound of sugar. I can and will draw on anything.

You want to dress up and act like different people or imagine your someone else? Not a clown that messes up and puts on a big red nose. I mean someone who has to act out all the time for attention. Not the ones that go "Blah, blah, blah," and "Honk, honk" goes the red nose.

So, why do I continue to bother you with my pettiness, when instead you ignore me, and I continue to bounce around like a happy clown?

Many times, it seems natural to put on a smiling face to appear to be someone different than who we really are. Most of the time the root of this is the fear of man—commonly known as peer pressure. The key here is to remember who you are in the Lord and walk in the realization that He is the only One we will ever have to give account to for the things we have either said or done.

So, the next time I want to act silly or clown around for attention, please remind me Lord that this is not who You called me to be and let me feel your peace. Let me remember Your peace because Your Words says in Isaiah 26:3, "You will keep him in perfect peace, whose mind is stayed on You, because he trusts in You."

Chapter Thirty-two

INNER BATTLE

It's so easy to smile and hide the fact that you are hurting.

It's so easy to fake your happiness in public and go home and cry.

It's easy to let people into your head and accept all the lies they claim you are.

I don't know. People just love to try to tear you down. The negativity has built up inside of me, and I don't know any other way to think.

I block people out because their words don't matter. I continue to have this fight with myself, so my life will never be right.

You ask yourself, "What's wrong with me? What did I do to deserve this? Do I deserve this? I must have done something to deserve this."

But I refuse.
I refuse to be your puppet.
I refuse to accept your lies.
I refuse to have a war with myself.

To let you take my happiness.

My joy.

My peace.

My love for life.

My confidence.

No more.

The fight with myself from listening to others has now ceased. Just as I mentioned in the "Clown" section, we can't please everyone all the time, and some we will never be able to please. However, the good news is, "We don't have to please them."

The peace that any of us needs only comes from the Father above. Once you step into His presence and experience His love and peace, you are changed forever. No longer do you battle with those inner thoughts. "You are the righteousness of God in Christ Jesus," according to His Word in 2 Corinthians 5:21, and everything within your soul helps you think and move forward on the path—the great path—He has chosen for you to follow.

Chapter Thirty-three

RACISM

Fury just burns inside of me like an open flame. Why are people so arrogant? So ignorant? Why does race matter? What makes me, a human being, any different from another? Skin color? That's weird.

As I previously mentioned, "What makes one crayon greater or less than the other? Can't both be used to create something beautiful?" Art can be pretty boring if it's only one shade. All of the famous artists were known because of their great creativity when it came to color. They understood the importance of blending the hues for an even greater work.

Why can't we do the same? Why can't we realize that every race plays a crucial part in what makes the world successful? Each culture is one crucial piece of the whole puzzle. Not all the pieces match, but when we work together, we create a beautiful picture. Once we realize that, we will live in a better, safer, more loveable earth.

You stereotype each other's races based on what?
Revenge?
Well, I want redemption, I want people to know we bleed the same color.

Racism disgusts me. There are false abuse claims. Why do you say my skin is so dark; honestly, does it matter … no tan lines? Hey, if you sat in the sun long enough, we all might be the same color.

A black man can't even be in a hurry to take his pregnant wife to the hospital without being racially profiled by a cop.

So, you're going to bump into me and act like you don't see me, as if I'm not standing here? I do deserve respect!

Inner racial couples are no longer safe, whether it's a white woman who is dating a black man or vice versa. People look at inner racial couples differently, as if they broke a law or something. They can't walk down the street together without stares or ugly words or judgement. This should be a place where mixed kids don't need protection.

How about we all become one race—the human race? Is it too much to want a better life, a peaceful life? I have to wonder how some of these same people will act when they get to Heaven (if they get to Heaven.) Every nationality will be represented there, and we will have perfect harmony. Well, if Jesus taught us to pray in the Lord's prayer, "Thy Kingdom come on earth, as it is in Heaven," (Matthew 6:10), wouldn't this be a part of that coming together, regardless of race or creed?

Through Christ our salvation includes loving our brother as ourselves. Maybe this is the real root of the problem. You can't love me because you don't love yourself. My heart goes out to you. God loves you. Please learn to accept his love and forgive yourself.

Let's walk in the love He gave us for one another so we can bring glory to God and fulfill His plan for mankind on earth.

Chapter Thirty-four

YOUR PROBLEM—
NOT MINE ... (ENEMIES)

You should control your life, not mine. Why do people blame other people for their problems? Or see others being a problem in their lives, instead of themselves?

People get so mad that you can't even control your feelings and your words.

I have looked out for you since day one, but our time has come to a close. I can no longer be attached to you, because I have changed, and so have you. We are in two different places in our lives, so now you call yourself cutting me off as I speak; you call me a liar. So why is it that I check on you, but you don't do that in return? Do you want to know that I'm safe too?

So, thank you for letting me know you are not as mature as I thought you were; that I have grown and you haven't.

Thank you for calling me out by name and letting me know how you really feel about me.

You say I never loved you, but we all know that's not true. Thanks for not listening at all to me, but more to yourself.

You only think of yourself. This is true because if I went down the list of what you did for me vs. what I did for you, there is no comparison that's even close.

You always ask me for help with doing things or giving you advice; but yet, you admitted to never using it or you twisted it around. So why waste my time? I tried to help you, but instead, you said I treated you like you were retarded. Well then, if you are retarded, so is everyone I talk to because nothing has changed about how I speak to people. You just knew at the time what you were going to do, and I was clueless.

I'm older, you're younger, what happened to respect for the older? And don't blame your parents or the way you grew up because at this point in your life you can teach yourself and read for yourself, so you should know better.

You even go to work and don't listen to those people so much that you have to ask me what to do when I know they told you how to access your files.

You claim you don't live paycheck to paycheck, but you don't like the job you are at because it's not a stable place. Yet, you complain about not having money. The last time I checked someone who wasn't living check to check wasn't complaining. Then you complain about not getting paid on time because you just started. Well, everyone knows when you're new, you are in the hole one week. My thing is this, if you have to complain so much, then that's not the job for you, boo.

So, now you are mad because people are talking about you or spreading lies. Who cares? Because you did it to others, so this is payback.

Now, who are you going to run to who will have your back the next time your attitude gets you in trouble? I'm not your enemy, and neither are they. You are your own enemy.

You asked me to spend time with you, but I work. I'm responsible, and mature people like me have their priorities straight. Hanging out is the last thing on the list because I'm not a teen anymore. I have bills to pay.

Of course, everyone makes time for what they want to make time for, and I need a place to live and a family to support.

Just know it's all about how you approach people when you want to talk to them, and you don't know how they may take the news, so watch the words you use so you might get a better outcome. People even feed off of your 'ora' because they can feel the negativity radiating off of you.

Just know if someone choked me, I wouldn't be trying to have a relationship with them, but it's your life. Do what you want because I am.

It's never my way or the highway, but I just know what I want and what I'm going to take or not take from others. It doesn't matter if I spend time with someone every week, every two months, or once a year. I don't love the person I see once a year any less than the person I saw yesterday. I honestly don't even have the energy to fight people in this world anymore. This is why people get killed every day for various reasons. Our attitude is one of the key ingredients that makes the difference.

You throw yourself a pity party and say your parents did you the same way. Well, that's not how I remember it happening. I actually remember you saying you ran away every time you had a problem. If it was with one person, you always wanted to bring in someone else to help you. Even then, not everyone will be on your side. It's not always in your favor.

Whatever the problem is, I know God will work it out, if we are willing to let Him. In the meantime, I can forgive you and love you, but it will be at a distance. Maybe we both need healing, but He is more than capable of doing it.

When offense comes, it's the work of the enemy. It's a trap from the devil himself, to see if we will get off of God's plan to walk in love and forgive others. I refuse to give someone that kind of power over me. Forgiveness isn't for the other person. Forgiveness is for me—to be free of any bondage or baggage that they are trying to create in my life. This doesn't excuse their wrong, but it keeps me free from living in the past. I can move into the present and receive all that God has for me each and every day.

Maybe this is why He says in His Word, "The path of the righteous gets brighter and brighter every day!" (Proverbs 4:18). Forgiving others is a foundational key to receiving that brighter path.

Chapter Thirty-five

OUR CHILDHOOD

Everyone has a very colorful childhood whether it's good for some or challenging for others. No matter what version your childhood was, that is what was planned for you since the day you were born.

Some people's childhood consists of learning to skate, riding bikes, playing outside in the dirt, climbing trees, taking naps, going to school and doing homework, playing with friends on playdates, playing dress up or having tea time, having water balloon fights, playing video games, eating lots of candy, sleeping countless hours in my bedroom or the back seat of the car or a random chair, or just being plain lazy, eating lots of food in order to grow, wanting to be grown because you couldn't have your way.

There was loving your siblings and having each other's backs, sitting in your parent's lap, and being picked up when you didn't feel like walking, birthday parties, getting whatever you wanted out of the store and not paying for it, playing at the park, or going swimming, learning right from wrong and getting in trouble for it, quality family meals and game nights, unexpected, all paid-for trips out of town, being happy because you learned how to do something for yourself, excited about the first day of school or when your first tooth fell out, being able to explore, taking field trips during school, coloring creating art, not having a care in the world, not being afraid to take risks, talking on the phone, wishing and dreaming about what you wanted to be when you grew up, sleepovers, and holidays together.

Why did we ever want to leave this place? I wish I could go back.

Don't forget your childhood village. It's important for us to remain grateful for our upbringing. In most families, sacrifices were made to provide not only the basic needs, but some of the wanted items as well. So, even if or when there were problems, we can thank God we made it through.

Now we are back to what the Word tells us in Psalm 136:1-3, "Give thanks to the LORD, for he is good. *His love endures forever.* Give thanks to the God of gods. *His love endures forever.* Give thanks to the Lord of lords: *His love endures forever.*"

Chapter Thirty-six

STARTING OVER

They say starting over isn't easy. But it's okay to start over. How dare you say that you don't want to do certain things because your "Ex" ruined it for you! Forget him!

How dare you say you are going to be lonely forever because love was ruined for you! Men have disrespected you so many times that you have lost hope inside, but you are fighting to find your prince charming, your Romeo. And if you were to try, you just don't know where to start, so you guard your heart and take a leap of faith.

You don't want to go to sporting events because that used to be your thing. Ya'll use to do that together and you can't let go yet, until you finally see someone fine, and now you can't wait until he comes to speak to you. Your eyes light up with excitement while talking to him, and your wall of fear disappears and you realize starting over isn't that hard, once you let go.

Starting over is okay even when your job becomes too much for you. It's ok to start over the interview process somewhere else. Who knows, this might be the window of opportunity for you to make more income. You must believe in yourself and know that you are an asset to anyone you meet, and you will succeed in everything you do.

Even when you say to yourself, "I just want to start over and do life again." I want you to know that this is not an option, but you can have a second chance to re-do some things you have done and change the outcome.

I ask you, "Why do we live our life in a circle, constantly repeating things when we don't have to?"

I know we all just want a better life, and please know, you can have it. However, the way to obtain something different lies within our thinking. If I continue to think or believe a certain thing, my actions or responses will remain the same. The Bible tell us in Proverbs 23:7, "As a man thinks in his heart, so is he."

So, if we want our situations to change, it is first necessary to change our thoughts … to renew our minds with the Word of God. The Word then says we will be "transformed by the Word" and not "conformed to the world" and our old way of thinking.

Chapter Thirty-seven

VENGEANCE

I want my redemption. I want to attack everyone around you that comes in my path. When will you grow up?

You'd rather be with people who continuously stab you in the back and beat up on you all the time, instead of being with the people who are always there for you—no matter what. The ones you should respect and who love you, you end up disrespecting the most—over and over again.

I ask you one question, then you attack me. So, I won't ask any more. I'm done. Having an attitude all the time isn't the answer, but you make me so angry.

I went out my way to help you and now for what? I can't even get a thank you from you. I just can't deal with you sometimes. You irritate me to no end.

Why do you steal from me? If you ask, I might just have given it to you.

When you learn life lessons, you need to apply them to the real world. But why would you? Because you don't care. You will push everyone around you away until you have no one left to love you. Then what are you going to do? Cause at this moment, I still don't like you, and I'm wondering what my payback is going to be.

The one person who tells you, I pay the bills, I own this house, I brought you into this world and I can take you out, you treat badly, as well.

So, when I try to talk to you, you're just going to ignore me now, and you know I don't like being ignored.

Do you think I work hard for nothing? Think again, you're going to be so mad once I reach the height of my goals and I am successful, and you're not invited to ride with me through this journey. I don't need a lying, stealing, cheating person in my life.

I thought I had changed my ways, and now you made me revert back to the old me. I don't like that. I don't like that I let you have that kind of power over me. Revenge is not the answer ...ever! In fact, the Bible makes it clear that revenge belongs to the Lord. He will pay them back. (Romans 12:19).

This should encourage us all that God is on our side, and He will bring things to light. He is a just God, and He takes care of His children.

Chapter Thirty-eight

LUST

I am looking at him, and I can hear him calling my name, but his lips are not even moving. My mind is in all types of bad places. The room is hot, or it could be just me. I have had a crush on you ever since I laid eyes on you, but I don't want to tell you because I think I may not be your type. I want to come and talk to you more than just the normal greetings we exchange, but I get nervous, and I might start saying things that may not make sense.

Overtime I look at you and you look at me. I look away with blushing cheeks and try to hold back a smile as I long for you. I want to just ask you to go out with me on a date, but I wait patiently for you to ask me. When you don't ask, I think that maybe you're afraid or just not man enough, so finally I get the nerve to say something and you shoot me down, which is okay.

I'm mature and it didn't hurt my feelings because now I know, but I still have a crush on you, and it's not going away. I think the excuse you gave me was wack, but it tells me you are not as mature as I am. Even though your looks may be appealing to me, we wouldn't be able to get along. I know because you would be acting childish.

My senses say that if you liked me enough you would change your ways. So, my friends say to me and tell me you are immature and that you like drama, which isn't my nature, and you still need time to grow up. Well at what age will you be before you decide to grow up ... 40 maybe?

The lust I have for you I wish was no more, but it is still knocking at my door. That's why I need my mind renewed to the Word. I need to focus on those thoughts like the Bible tells us in Philippians 4:8, "Finally, brothers and sisters, whatever is true, whatever is noble, whatever is right, whatever is pure, whatever is lovely, whatever is admirable—if anything is excellent or praiseworthy— think about such things."

When I think about these things, you don't come to mind. I'm free of any of the unhealthy desires and I have peace. Thank You, God.

Chapter Thirty-nine

THE OPPOSITE PERSON

When you first meet someone, you are getting to know them because you have to learn the real true them. But over a course of months, the person you know is not the person you remember them being.

They always say random things, treat you bad, or have negative things to say about someone, but that's not the person because you know them, too.

They're the totally opposite of what you were thinking. You have the man vs. the little boy, or the woman vs. the young girl. They set you up, they lie, they retaliate, they have you asking, who are they really?

Then you say something to them, and they ask you, "Who am I to you or who do you think I am?" Uh oh. Do you tell the truth or tell them what they want to hear? Then you get hit with the attitude statement: "You don't really know me, do you?" You're shocked. You realize they're not all there. They may even need a check-up.

They yell and scream, but you blanked out and didn't hear anything, because you know they think you're crazy for being with them.

I mean they say you are who you hang with. It's like you were just hit with the two faces of drama—the one is happy and the other is sad. You're confused and a little scared.

Allow me to help you, and I'm going to tell you, you should cut them loose. Many times, we even stay in relationships because we think we might be able to help others. However, the truth is, before it's all over, we can become as mentally unbalanced as they are. Amos 3:3 in the Bible makes this clear. "How can two walk together unless they are agreed or in unity?"

This is when it's important to ask the Holy Spirit for direction and follow what He says to do in your friendships. He will lead you and guide you in all truth, so we can trust Him and keep healthy relationships as part of the benefits of having our relationship with Him.

Chapter Forty

UNCERTAINTY

Have you ever been in a season in your life where it seems like too much is happening at the same time, and it seems really hard to handle and process it all? If not, the time will come. It's a weird time, honestly. It is extremely hard to not lose your own self in return to worrying about everything else around you.

Imagine your life as a plastic plate and suddenly the cafeteria lady slams on a glob of mashed potatoes and meat. Suddenly, you feel the plate start to bend, and you have this anxiety that it will break—no matter how you hold it, or the food could even slide off on the floor. You will never know how something that heavy could stand on something that is labeled so light. It is not logically or statistically able to hold all this weight and not bend or break, but somehow it does.

In a sense, that plate could be any of us at any point in our lives, both young and old. The odds are definitely not in our favor—when it seems like too much is happening at the same time, and it seems really hard to handle and process it all. If it's not now, the time will come. It's a strange time, not losing who you are in exchange for worrying about everything else around you.

But just like that plate, if we just hold on, we can be amazed at how much weight we can hold.

This is why Jesus instructed us to not worry. Yes, He said there would be trials and tribulation, but to be of good cheer. Why? Because He had overcome the troubles in the world. (John 16:33).

Now I know that doesn't seem to make any sense when there are still so many problems, but this is when we have to remind ourselves that He has it all under control. How do we do this? By ...

"...fixing our eyes on Jesus, the pioneer (author) and perfecter (finisher) of faith. For the joy set before him he endured the cross, scorning its shame, and sat down at the right hand of the throne of God. Consider him who endured such opposition from sinners, so that you will not grow weary and lose heart" (Hebrews 12:2-3, NIV).

Regardless of what it may look like around us, if we keep our eyes on Him, the Author and Finisher of our faith, we will always be victorious. Thank You, Lord!

Chapter Forty-one

A LETTER TO MY ALOPECIA FRIENDS

Thank you for showing me how to approach defying the odds of life and that strength comes from more than just what you look like. When I thought that I couldn't go on anymore because I looked ugly, when I looked at you ... you gave me strength.

People look at us and say, "Oh, you don't look sick," and some people stare.

I try to cover my flaws as best as I can. But you let your inner beauty shine bright. Seeing that made me stronger than those can even imagine.

Know we are uniquely beautiful.

As my hair continues to shed, my eyebrows and lashes fall away, I'm no longer saddened, but encouraged. All thanks to you.

Know there is a way to make us feel whole again.

There is so much in store for you and me. So much more than to be worried about than our outer appearance. Our hair is not what makes us who we are. It's what's inside of us.

Just know the beauty in you and me is flawless. Our skin radiates, and we are the image of true perfection.

Revelation 4:11 says, "You are worthy, our Lord and God, to receive glory and honor and power, for you created all things, and by your will they were created and have their being."

God created us—uniquely—because He loves variety and beauty. He created mankind in His image. So, why should I be focused on only the exterior when He created me to be like Him?

Chapter Forty-two

THE BACKSTABBER

I turn my back to you in order to show you the major huge knife and other knives you stabbed me with. So, in that case we do not need a conversation. Why do you lie about me continuously?

You say I was rude to you.
You say I bullied you.
You say I yelled at you.
You say I ignored you.
You say I don't want to work with you.
You said I told you to do the opposite of what management told you, and instead you listened to me.

Everything you said is all untrue. In reality, all I did was ask you a question about the work we were supposed to be doing together. You felt a certain way because you thought I was questioning your authority or trying to undermine you or talking at you because you think I'm better than you.

You change the story on what actually happened every time I talk to you. Did I actually say or do these things to you for you to treat me this way?

No, so is it because you are intimidated by me, that you make up things to report on me? Honestly, you irritate me because the things you are doing are childish, petty, and stupid. Now you are not even cooperating with me because you feel a certain type of way. Your sending emails to everyone but me, and when someone asks me a question, I'm clueless about what they're speaking of.
I get angry because I really want to get an attitude with you and rip a few bad words your way, but I choose to stay professional.

Now there are all these rumors about me. The rumors have everyone talking about one another to me, and now I'm wondering who do I really trust and where is all this information coming from? The bosses ask me questions, and I know they hear things, but they aren't sure what to do because something isn't right with the whole situation.

So when I say something, they tell me no matter what you have a job, but yet I show up to work one morning locked out and my credentials don't work. I call and they inform me that someone inputted that my last day was yesterday. I'm confused. I find out later it was an error, but who created the error. I'm the nicest, calmest person here, but yet, you want to stab a knife through my back. I'm not the one talking bad about you. I only listen.

If you only asked me questions, I would have told you the answers you seek, but don't accuse me of something

110

I didn't do nor say. I'm not the bad guy here … you are. Especially when you don't show up for a week, claiming you're sick when someone said they saw you in public and another said they even spoke to you and you didn't look sick to them. They said you weren't coughing or that you looked miserable—actually you seemed like your normal self. You've lied so much now people are whispering and not believing you.

The one thing I've learned about a person who lies to me is … they're not just lying to me. Sooner or later they get caught in the web of lies they tell. The saddest part is, after they have told the lies for so long, I don't believe they even know in reality what the truth really is. This is a bad situation for everyone now.

Even though it may be necessary to work with these kind of individuals, you have to realize how emotionally unstable they really are. The Bible is very clear about praying for our enemies or those who willingly persecute you. (Matthew 5:44). Is this easy? Absolutely not, but if our Lord and Savior could ask His Father to forgive those who crucified Him, we should be able to forgive those around us, as well. Just remember, He works all things for our good. (Romans 8:28).

Chapter Forty-three

OVERQUALIFIED CANDIDATE

I went to high school and graduated with a Diploma. I went to college and graduated with a bachelor's degree. I went to trade school and graduated with a certificate. I take continuing education classes to learn new things to keep up with the changing times.

I have so much knowledge that I could possibly run a company or become an asset for yours. Yet, it's hard for me to find a job. Why do they say I'm overqualified? Some even say underqualified or they don't think I can handle the job.

I have the Perfect resume, perfect cover letter, and I can do these requirements:

> Oversee and Delegate employees
> Process Mail
> Organize or set up a Website
> Schedule appointments
> Book travel arrangements
> Payroll processing
> Support or Promote Guidelines
> Work closely with safety and security, regarding
>   management/procedures for safety
> Monitor daily activity

Create lesson plans for schools
Cash handle for sales
Keep records and information
Help colleagues with routine administrative work
Use and fix office equipment, such as fax
    machines and photocopiers, etc.
Respond to questions and provide information
Type, format, proofread, and edit correspondence
    and other documents
Manage multiple schedules, calendars and
    arrange appointments
Use computers for spreadsheet, word processing,
    database management, and other
    applications
Greet walk-in customers, other visitors, and
    escort them to specific destinations
Organization Management of Office
Monitor Daily activity of classroom
Provide classroom management
Ensure every students' academic success
Align every activity with the districts core beliefs
Administer CPR and first aid
Graphic designer

My success is much greater than my failures.

So, even if I'm overqualified, I'd rather have something
than nothing, which is the situation I am currently in. Let
me work for you!

When we find ourselves in situations like this one, faith is what sustains us. Knowing that the God and creator of this world loves you and has a great plan for you is comforting. Even as the "Waymaker" song states, *"Even when I don't see it, You're working ... even when I don't feel it, You're working ... You are always working."*

Philippians 2:13 says, "... for it is God who works in you to will and to act in order to fulfill his good purpose." At times like these we must trust in God. Use our faith— stand on our faith. He will make every good and perfect thing come to pass in our lives!

Chapter Forty-four

THE ONLY CHILD

Being the only child stinks from the beginning to the end. There is no one for you to play with. No one to share stories or secrets with. There is no one to get in trouble with or blame things on, so that you are not in trouble.

There are always adults around, and you hear things, but when you repeat it, they get mad, even though they said it first. How were you supposed to know not to repeat it as a child? If I hadn't been in a room full of adults, I never would have heard it; plus, I could have been playing with someone my own age, if I was able to have playdates or sleepovers.

Being an only child does make you grow up fast anyway, especially if your parents are older because they were old when they had you. So, before you hit 18, it is your job to be responsible for a lot—like making sure the house chores are taken care of and that we don't need groceries, etc.

As a young person you are so stressed because you are taking on roles that should be done by someone over 21, better yet, 25 years of age, and you're only 16.

And don't let your parents get sick or go to the hospital. You have to figure out how to get medicine, how to make sure they are cared for, if you are away, calling everyone to inform them of the situation, etc.

The hardest thing to face as an only child is death. Not knowing where to start because your emotions of sadness and fear are so high.

But then again it does have its advantages—like when you were a child and you got any and everything you wanted. Not having to share.

Now, as an older person, I get all the attention, gifts, and the monetary items are all mine—no one else's. Parents support anything I want. But what can I say ... these are the problems of an only child.

These feelings were changed and also comforted when I learned that I had a Heavenly Father. My earthly family may go to Heaven one day, but the God of Heaven would be with me always ... here and now ... and forever. Thank You, God, for always being there for me. I know I have nothing to fear. "I am" never alone because the great "I AM" is with me. Hallelujah!

Chapter Forty-five

THE "EX"

Have you been with someone that you wish you had never met? The person who you thought you would be with for life, but it just didn't pan out the way you expected. The person who would say, "I love you," and you would say it back. I was love stricken by you. I now know I was blind.

You know, I am the one who helped you get to the platform you are sitting on today. I am the one who drove you to higher limits you didn't see yourself on because I wanted you to be better for me, but yet I made you better for someone else. I dimmed my worth for you, and you wasted my time. Did you even think or know what I am worth? Or was it all about you? Even though I knew that you were not treating me for what I was worth—I stayed.

I'm frustrated to say the least.

My curiosity wonders. Your discombobulated mind has trapped me, and I honestly thought we could have an opposites attraction due to you being an introvert and me an extrovert. I thought about how if we both don't mean the same to each other, then we are not one another's best friend.

119

You are withdrawn from this life if you think you are the only one who will get what they want from life. You want someone to feel sympathetic for you, and I no longer will. I do not approve of your actions. You were so aggressive, and yet I stayed. You know, listening skills are important, and you didn't utilize it well. When you don't listen, it makes people feel less important, but I even overlooked that. You actually belittled me at times, and I got over it.

When I love, I love hard, with my whole heart, and you took my love. When I tried to give my love, it was abused and misused. I'm sorry for both of our losses. Our marriage could have been a success. You could have been my love, my best friend. We could have been a power couple, pushing each other to accomplish everything.

We could have had it all because of God's covenant plans for marriage. The Word says in Ecclesiastes 4:9, "Two are better than one because they have a good return for their labor: If either of them falls down, one can help the other up..." I thank God that now He is my helper!

Chapter Forty-six

YOUR OPINIONS

Let me tell you a thing or two about your opinions—your unwanted, unasked for opinions. Your opinions don't matter, because at the end of the day, I'm going to do what is best for me and my life. I do not care about your opinions. Your opinions are like sardines (they stink), and I don't care for them.

You give me your opinion, and then see me and ask me, "How did it go?" I tell you, "Great," and you ask, "What did you do? Did you take my advice?" I tell you, "No."

Now, just a moment ago you were happy that you thought your opinion was taken into consideration, but when I told you I succeeded anyway, without doing what you thought I should do, your whole attitude changes. Why is that? My life is not your life, and I can think for myself. My world doesn't revolve around your world or what you say. So, get over yourself. When I want your help, advice, or opinion, trust me, I will ask for it.

I'm tough on myself, and the problem is I set a standard for myself and I hold everyone around me to the same standard. They always disappoint me.

I'm driven to obtain my goals on my own without your unwanted opinions. You just don't know when to quit or when enough is enough because now you insult me and say mean things to me.

Opinions are overrated! Yes, advice is good at times if it is just that ... advice. If not, it comes in the form of control and manipulation, which creates fear—fear of man— peer pressure to have to follow someone else's ideas or thoughts, rather than being able to stand up for what you think or believe is the right thing for your own life.

The Bible says the counsel of many is using wisdom. Proverbs 15:22 says, "Plans fail for lack of counsel, but with many advisers they succeed." The key to this is: Who are your counselors or advisors? The best Counselor any of us have is the Holy Spirit. Jesus Himself said it was better for Him to go so the Spirit of God could come. (John 16:7). One of the many things the Spirit does is lead us and guide us into all truth. AND He knows us better than we know ourselves (Romans 8:27) ... so why wouldn't we ask Him for directions or advice? Our answers will be sure when we ask and trust God. He knows who we can trust for help while we are on earth.

Chapter Forty-seven

EXCUSES

Excuses make me cringe.
Excuses are for losers, people that don't dream or have ambition.
Excuses are for the weak-willed person.
Excuses are for the lazy couch-potato person.
Excuses are for those people who want to be given everything and work for nothing.
Excuses make me angry.
Excuses lie—telling you because you are not happy you can run and quit.
Excuses say you have no compassion for my struggles.
That you are the epitome of an angry black woman. Don't you know we fight to make that stern type disappear. I won't let you get to me or under my skin or take my power with your excuses.

Sorry, but excuses are not welcome here.

Truthfully, they are just another form of blaming some "one" or some "thing" for our lack of responsibility—or our lack of whatever.

The sad part about excuses is if we never accept our part in anything, then how do we ever fix it? Not only in how it relates to others, but especially in our own lives. If it's never my fault, then how can I ask God to forgive me so I can be free to move forward? So I can have peace in a situation that maybe didn't turn out so well?

We all make mistakes—miss the mark—as the Word calls it. However, when we own up to it and ask God to forgive us, He is not only quick to forgive, but He also tosses it into the sea of forgetfulness. (Hebrews 8:12; Micah 7:18). This is what gives us the power to overcome sin and live a victorious life in Him.

Chapter Forty-eight

THE BUSY LIFE

I can't complain of this life because I asked for it, but what about you? I'm busy cause I'm broke. I refuse to be a statistic, as the world says I should be. They say I should be living paycheck to paycheck. They say I should be helping others live out their dreams, but what about my dreams, and who should be helping me. I'm busy because I want to be.

Would I like to have the picture-perfect life? Yes, but that isn't the life I was born into. I can't just go on an impromptu vacation when I want to. I have to work. I work from 7 a.m. to 11 p.m., and then I still have to find time to clean my house, do the dishes, wash my clothes and iron them, grocery shop and then cook, so I can eat, and pay bills. All of this must repeat itself every week Monday through Sunday.

Oh, and let's not forget I have to find time to have a personal life, which is spending time with the kids, hanging out with friends and going on dates. I can honestly say I utilize very hour I have in life to my fullest potential, but through it all, I do find time to rest. Sometimes, a girl just wants to sit down and watch TV until my eyelids can't stay open anymore, and I end up in the other universe just for a few hours to wake up and do it all over again.

Some days I sleep in my car because I don't have the strength to muster up to get out of the car to go inside the house. Power naps are great, but that's not me. I work hard so I can rest with no worries.

People ask me, "Why do I work like I'm the last person on earth, trying to recreate life and living?" I work hard so I can play hard.

They say, "You need to eat." Eat … that's not on the schedule. "You need to go home and go to sleep, especially if you don't feel well." Sleep, no thank you. I will do that when my time comes to go to Heaven.

I got so much going on that you are confused about life and what you are doing. What you need to do is slow down.

I live the busy bee life. However, I've now come to recognize my priorities. Once I decided to put God first, I could rest in the fact that He has promised me certain things as His child. Does this mean I just sit back and don't work? Of course not, but I don't have the pressure on me anymore that, "I'm out here by myself. If I don't do it, no one will."

I have His promise through the covenant He established with me that every good and perfect gift comes from above—it comes from my Father. (James 1:17). And in Revelation 3:7 it is written, "To the angel of the church in Philadelphia write: These are the words of him who is holy and true, who holds the key of David. What he opens no one can shut, and what he shuts no one can open."

In other words, I know God has my front and my back. My footsteps are ordered by Him, and I will move forward in victory because of it.

Chapter Forty-nine

ACCIDENT PRONE

Why do you keep getting hurt? Are you hurting yourself? Why are you the magnet for incidents? Why must you continue to call me and stress me out every week with this, and I have to come and save you?

I don't understand why you want to stress me out with your life, as if I don't have my own issues to deal with and want no extra part of yours.

Why do you refuse to go to the hospital when you are bleeding from your head?

Then help me understand how you forgot what you said just that fast. This is how I know you're hurt. You say you don't try to hurt yourself on purpose. I believe you—I do. You say the cabinet fell apart and it fell on you. How? Did you slam it?

Here we go again. You hurt yourself and you are bleeding, but you won't go and get stitches.

Do you always have to tell me your life story every time I see you? I feel like this is your way of trying to throw me off course of making you go to the hospital.

As soon as you think you are healed or every time you go back to work, you go back to doing random things like moving furniture, gardening in the yard, and doing DIY projects.

As I know this, I do stay prepared for my phone to ring in order for me to come and help you, since you are so stubborn. I guess I'm the only help you are willing to get, and I will be there for your accident-prone self.

However, God has given us many verses in His Word to use as our shield against such things. We should be declaring these verses in advance for protection.

Psalm 91:11, "For He will give His angels charge concerning you, To guard you in all your ways."

Isaiah 54:17, " No weapon formed against you will prosper …"

Psalm 5:12, "Surely, LORD, you bless the righteous; you surround them with your favor as with a shield."

Philippians 4:19, "And my God will supply every need of yours according to his riches in glory in Christ Jesus."

Chapter Fifty

THE MIRACLE CHILD

Have you ever been told you couldn't be pregnant? Yet, you always wanted a family of your own. Even though you know there are adoption and surrogacy options, it's just not the same for you, when you want to experience something of your own.

They said I couldn't have a child. They said there was no way, but I never believed them. I continued to live my life as if it would always just be me and no littles ones. Until the day the one I always dreamed of having is finally here.

Now your whole world has changed, and it has been flipped upside down. You now have to think of not only yourself, but someone else. You now have to care for the one you always wanted and waited for. The one you want to call your little best friend. The one you now get to mentor and teach things to because you never had that growing up, and you wish you had had someone there for you.

You realize your wish of having someone to love unconditionally has come true, and I say to my miracle child, "I can't wait to meet you!"

This experience just reminds us of how much our Heavenly Father loves us. The Word states, "He knew us before we were ever formed in our mother's womb" (Jeremiah 1:5). His love for us was so great that He was willing to let His own child, Jesus, die for our sins, so we could be restored and united into His family again. No greater love is there than this.

Chapter Fifty-one

HOARDER

Why must you have an attachment to everything? It is not as important as it may seem. If you part ways with it you may feel freer, instead of feeling weighed down endlessly.

Not being able to walk through the room without things falling over or are in your way. Being unable to find the one thing you are looking for. I honestly don't think you realize how much stuff you have.

You panic when you think something is missing. Why do you have an attachment to unnecessary things? You can give me the reason on why every item is here, but maybe it's time to let go of the reason and the season that belongs to that item. The more you let go, the better you will feel.

You claim you have everything you need, but when is too much ... too much ... instead of having just enough?

All I see is junk staring at me. From old magazines, newspapers, books, clothes, broken furniture, pillows, old electronics, papers after papers of bills and mail, decorations, pictures, plastic bags, boxes, and so much more. I mean too much more.

The hoarder in you will not trap itself in me. So here, let me help set you free.

I bet you wish I would mind my own business, but just know you are my business and my hot mess.

But I am blessed to have you, and so I come to save you. I come to help you see that our worth and value is not tied up in the material things that are around us. In fact, the Word asks, "What profits a man if he gains the whole world, but loses his soul?" (Mark 8:36). The soul is our mind, will and emotions. If we become so tied down to our possessions emotionally that we can't part with anything, and our homes look like the junkyard, full of bugs and unhealthy debris, is that not a form of losing our minds—insanity?

At some point, we will leave it all behind, for none of us can take anything with us after our life on earth ends. Let us prepare for that journey today … both spiritually and in the natural.

Chapter Fifty-two

RANDOM THOUGHTS

My mind races and wonders. Sometimes, I can't stop it from overthinking or running into nowhere land.

Why don't I have a relationship? But why have a relationship when you have friends—who do the same things for you, like get on my nerves, talk too late at night, etc.?

How people bite off the hand that was helping them. Guess what? You need me before I will ever need you. Do you think it is okay to talk to me any kind of way? Or why do you continue to cut me off while I'm speaking? So then you and I are not cool anymore, and this you know, but yet you see me and walk up behind me and make a smart comment, like you wanted me to respond.

I'm bigger than that, which is your childish immature ways. I saw you and heard you, but I choose not to entertain you. So, yes, I ignore you because I value peace rather than drama.

I just think how you took my inexperience in certain areas or my niceness and used it to your advantage.

I think about how movies and news can corrupt peoples' minds because it gives them ideas of things to do, which is why we have so many bad outcomes. When someone thinks up crazy things for a movie, I don't think they imagine someone would actually do this in real life.

I think about how every time I try to get ahead in life there is always something that shows up out of the blue to push me backwards or slows down my process or my goals.

I think about how I don't understand why teens are always on their phones, but they can't answer it or call you back when you know they have a missed call or they are logged into social media.

These are the reasons why I can't sleep because my brain is on overload all the time.

There will always be things that try to steal our peace. This is one of the things the enemy was sent to do … "steal, kill and destroy." Jesus Himself said in John 10:10, "The thief comes only to steal and kill and destroy; I have come that they may have life, and have it to the full." The way to rest our minds and allow peace to take charge is to stay in God's Word. When we meditate on His goodness to us, we will find peace and rest.

Chapter Fifty-three

COUNTRY LIFE

Have you ever been in the country just to get away and have time to unwind? The things I love about the country are: Quiet time to think
Horseback riding
ATV riding
Trail rides
Sitting on the porch, watching the sun rise and set
Playing hide and seek
Shucking peas
Eating mudbugs
Milking cows
Tending the chickens and chasing them around
Going fishing
Road trips to nearby towns
Playing in the dirt
Going swimming
Making mud pies
Walking for miles just to visit family
Having family reunions.

Living the country life is a great life. If you've never been, you should visit. God created the heavens and the earth. (Genesis 1:1). When you visit these places, look for His handiwork. Trust me, you will see it and be amazed!

MEET THE AUTHOR

April Brewer is a native of Dallas, Texas. *Greyed* is her debut novel.

April received her Bachelor's of Science Degree in Business Administration from Kaplan University after attending Cedar Valley College and Texas Southern University for a short time.

She works in the field of healthcare and is passionate about helping others and making life better for herself and her dad.

She is a single, female Christian, who talks a lot.

www.ingramcontent.com/pod-product-compliance
Lightning Source LLC
Chambersburg PA
CBHW050728030426
42336CB00012B/1462